Copyright 2023

Table of Contents

Arthritis is an inflammation of the joints. It can affect one joint or multiple joints. There are more than Trusted Source 100 different types of arthritis, with different causes and treatment methods.

Osteoarthritis (OA) is the most common type of arthritis Trusted Source in the United States. Other common types Trusted Source include:

Rheumatoid arthritis (RA)

Psoriatic arthritis (PsA)

Gout

The symptoms of arthritis usually develop over time, but they may also appear suddenly. The typical age for developing rheumatoid arthritis (RA) is between ages 30 and 50. It can, however, affect children, teens, and younger adults.

Osteoarthritis (OA) commonly develops after the age 50 or 60 years, but there are studies that reveal radiographic evidence of OA occurring in women in their 40s. It also tends to be more prevalent in individuals who are overweight.

BREAKFAST

1. Crustless Mini Quiche (Single Serving Breakfast Muffins)

Prep Time: 10 Minutes

Cook Time: 25 Minutes

Servings: 12-16

Ingredients

Base:

- 12 large eggs
- ½ cup heavy cream
- ¼ cup milk
- 2 TBSP fresh parsley, chopped
- 2 TBSP fresh basil, chopped (or other herb)
- ¼ tsp. salt
- ¼ tsp. pepper

Veggies:

- 1 cup broccoli, cut into teeny tiny florets
- 1 cup fresh spinach, roughly chopped
- 1 red bell pepper, chopped small
- ¼-1/2 cup onion, diced fine
- 1 jalapeno pepper, seeds and veins removed, diced fine (optional)
- Add-ins (optional):
- 1½ cups cheddar, gruyere, mozzarella, or other cheese, divided
- 1 lb. bacon, sausage, or other meat, fully cooked

Instructions

1. If using meat (bacon, sausage, etc.), cook it fully first. Set it aside to cool, then cut into small pieces.
2. Preheat oven to 375 degrees F., and thoroughly grease (butter, coconut oil, or non-stick spray) a muffin tin. (NOTE: I recommend using a non-stick muffin tin for even easier removal.)
3. In a large bowl, whisk together the eggs, cream, milk, parsley, basil, salt, and pepper. Set aside.
4. Get all your veggies diced up and ready to go. Optionally, you can saute your onion with a bit of olive oil to soften it up and take away some of its bite. Set aside and allow to cool.
5. Add all the veggies to the bowl with the egg mixture, and stir to combine. Stir in half of the cheese, and all of the meat, if using.
6. Using an ice-cream scoop or ¼ cup measure, scoop the mixture into the prepared muffin pan. Fill to about ¼ inch from the top, then sprinkle a small amount of reserved cheese over each. Place in the oven, and bake for 20-25 minutes, or until the egg is fully set and the cheese has just started to turn golden on top.
7. Remove from the oven and let cool for 5-10 minutes before running a butter knife around each muffin, and gently removing from the pan. Enjoy while warm, or let cool completely before storing in an airtight container in the fridge. Leftovers can be reheated for several seconds in the microwave (time will vary depending on your microwave), or a few minutes in a preheated oven or toaster oven.

Prep Time: 35 Minutes

Cook Time: 50 Minutes

Servings: 5

Ingredients

Tomatoes:

- 4 medium vine tomatoes
- 4 rashers streaky bacon (we use Freedom Farms)
- 4 toothpicks
- Omelettes:
- 8 eggs
- 3 tablespoons finely chopped basil or flat-leaf parsley
- sea salt and freshly ground pepper

To Serve:

- 2-3 cured chorizo sausages
- handful of rocket leaves
- grilled bread
- tomato chutney

Instructions

1. Preheat the oven to 180°C.
2. Tomatoes: Wrap each tomato in a rasher of bacon and secure with a toothpick. Place on a baking tray and drizzle with a little olive oil, salt and pepper. Bake for 8-10 minutes until the bacon is cooked.

3. Cut the chorizo into 3-4 long pieces. Heat a little olive oil in a sauté pan and cook the chorizo until golden. Drain on kitchen towels and keep warm in a low oven.

4. Omelettes: Break 2 eggs into a small dish and whisk in a ¼ of the herbs and season. Heat a 26 cm sauté pan with a little olive oil over a medium heat and pour in the eggs. Tilt the pan to distribute the eggs evenly and cook for 1 minute or until just set. Flip the omelet over and cook the other side briefly. Slide onto a plate and keep warm while you make the remaining omelets.

5. To serve: Spread each omelet with tomato chutney and top with chorizo and rocket. Fold in the sides and transfer to plates. Serve with the bacon-wrapped tomatoes, grilled bread and extra tomato relish.

Prep Time: 35 Minutes

Cook Time: 45 Minutes

Servings: 6

Ingredients

- 1 cup black quinoa (you could use white quinoa)
- 2 cups vegetable or chicken stock
- 4 free-range eggs (can be increased to 2 eggs per person)
- 150 grams baby kale leaves, rocket or mixed greens
- extra-virgin olive oil, for drizzling
- 1 avocado, cut into slices
- 3 radishes, cut into wafer thin slices
- sauerkraut, allow about ¼ cup per person (I used the Be Nourished brand)
- 200 grams haloumi cheese
- oil for frying
- 1 lemon, cut into wedges
- ground black pepper

To Garnish:

- micro-greens or sprouts, sesame seeds and fresh mint leaves

Instructions

1. Rinse the quinoa well under running water using a fine sieve. Place in a saucepan with the stock. Bring to a boil before reducing to a simmer. Cook with a lid slightly

ajar for 15–20 minutes until tender and the stock has been absorbed. Let sit for 5 minutes with the lid on.

2. Bring another saucepan of water to a boil and carefully lower the eggs in. Cook for 6 minutes for soft-boiled eggs. Run under cold water and peel.

3. Divide the quinoa and greens between 4 bowls or plates. Drizzle with olive oil. Top with the avocado, radish and sauerkraut. Halve the eggs and place on top.

4. Cut haloumi into 5mm slices. Heat a couple of spoonful of oil in a sauté pan over a medium to high heat. Cook the haloumi for 1 minute on each side until golden brown.

5. Place on top of the salad with lemon wedges for squeezing. Garnish with micro-greens, sesame seeds, fresh mint leaves and a generous grind of black pepper.

Prep Time: 15 Minutes

Cook Time: 20 Minutes

Servings: 8

Ingredients

Dry ingredients:

- 3 cups (380g.) all-purpose flour, plus more for dusting
- ⅓rd cup (76g.) sugar
- 2 tsp. baking powder
- ½ tsp. baking soda
- ½ tsp. salt
- 6 TBSP (3oz.) unsalted butter, cold and cut into cubes
- 7 oz. almond paste, frozen (I used this one)
- ¾ cup fresh cranberries, rinsed and dried

Wet ingredients:

- 1 large egg
- ¾ cup milk, or almond milk
- 1 tsp. lemon juice (can substitute white vinegar if you want)
- ½ tsp. almond extract
- ½ tsp. vanilla extract

For the top:

- 1-2 TBSP milk, for brushing
- 3-5 TBSP sliced almonds
- 1-2 TBSP coarse sugar

Instructions

1. Preheat oven to 400 degrees F., and line a baking sheet with parchment paper, or a silpat.
2. In a large bowl, whisk together the first five dry ingredients (the flour to the salt). Add the cubed butter, and cut it into the flour with a pastry cutter (or, transfer everything to a food processor and pulse a few times) until the butter is in pea-sized chunks.
3. Grate the almond paste on the large-hole side of a box grated. Using your fingers, gently mix the shreds into the dry ingredients so each one is separate and coated with flour. Mix in the cranberries.
4. In a separate bowl, whisk together the wet ingredients. Add the dry to the wet, and stir until everything is just evenly combined.
5. Sprinkle some flour on your cutting board or counter, and turn the dough out of the bowl. Gently shape the dough into a mound, and pat the mound into a disc about 1 inch thick. (If you want to make twice as many smaller scones, you can split the dough in half and make two smaller discs.)
6. Brush the top with milk, and sprinkle evenly with sliced almonds and sugar -- I like to gently pat the almonds into the top of the dough to make sure they stick. Using a long knife, divide the dough into 8 even triangles (like you would a pie).
7. Place each scone on your prepared baking sheet, leaving at least 1 inch of space between them. Bake on the center rack for about 18-20 minutes, or until the tops are lightly golden brown. (If you made smaller scones, reduce the baking time and keep a close eye on them.)
8. Let cool for 5-10 minutes before digging in. Scones are best eaten right away, while they are still a little warm

and lightly crisp at the edges, but they will keep well for up to 4-5 days. Once completely cool, store in an airtight container at room temperature. Serve as is, or with a dollop of whipped cream, cream fraiche, or clotted cream.

Prep Time: 35 Minutes

Cook Time: 25 Minutes

Servings: 4

Ingredients

- 500 grams Brussels sprouts, thinly shaved with a mandolin or very thinly sliced
- 6 kale leaves, stems removed, very thinly sliced
- 6 free-range eggs
- 1 cup finely grated parmesan, to sprinkle
- Sea salt and ground pepper
- Tempeh Bacon
- ¼ cup olive oil
- 4 teaspoons tamari
- ¼ teaspoon hot smoked paprika
- 1 teaspoon liquid smoke (optional but recommended)
- 2 tablespoons brown sugar
- ½ teaspoon ground cumin
- 250 grams tempeh

Croutons:

- 3 thick slices rye sourdough bread, torn into chunks
- Oil, to drizzle

Caesar Dressing:

- 5 anchovies, I used Ortiz
- 1 clove garlic
- Juice 1 lemon
- ½ cup good-quality mayonnaise

- ½ cup finely grated parmesan
- Ground pepper
- Vegan Caesar Dressing
- ½ cup good-quality
- Vegan mayonnaise
- ½ teaspoon grain mustard
- 1 small garlic clove, finely diced
- Juice ½ lemon

Instructions

1. Tempeh Bacon: Whisk together the olive oil, tamari, paprika, liquid smoke, sugar and cumin. Cut the tempeh lengthways into strips that are roughly ½ cm thick. Place in a shallow dish and drizzle over the marinade. Refrigerate for 4–24 hours.
2. Preheat the oven to 180°C.Line an ovenproof dish with baking paper and lay out the tempeh slices. Bake for 20 minutes, turning once halfway through. They can be used warm or stored in the fridge and used cold.
3. Croutons: Preheat the oven to 160°C.
4. Drizzle the bread with oil and season generously. Bake for 25 minutes. Can be made up to 4 hours in advance. If storing, allow to cool completely before placing in an airtight container.
5. Caesar Dressing: Combine the anchovies and garlic in a mortar and pestle. Pound until a smooth paste forms. Add the remaining ingredients and season with pepper to taste.
6. Vegan Caesar Dressing: Combine ingredients and season.

7. To Assemble: Combine the brussels sprouts and kale with the dressing of your choice and mix well. It's ideal to let the dressing soften the salad for 10 minutes.
8. Bring a medium saucepan of water to a boil. Carefully drop in the eggs. Cook for 6 minutes. Remove from the heat, run under cold water and peel carefully. Cut in half.
9. Divide the salad between 4 plates. Top with the eggs, tempeh bacon, croutons and parmesan. Serve immediately.

Prep Time: 35 Minutes

Cook Time: 25 Minutes

Servings: 4

Ingredients

- 250 grams good quality ready rolled puff pastry
- 1 egg whisked with 2 teaspoons milk or cream
- 150 grams chevre or soft goat cheese
- 16 spears asparagus, trimmed, halved lengthways and through the center
- 4 eggs, preferably free range organic
- 80 grams prosciutto
- sea salt and freshly ground black pepper
- finely grated zest of 1 lemon
- 2 tablespoons finely chopped chives

Instructions

1. Preheat the oven to 200°C and line an oven tray with baking paper. Cut the puff pastry into 4 equal pieces and place on the oven tray.
2. Gently mark a 1cm border around the edge of each piece of pastry to cut just half way through. Brush the edges with a little of the egg wash and use the tines of a fork to gently prick the inside base of each pastry square (Make at least 8–9 prick marks).

3. Bake for 10 minutes, then remove from the oven and poke down all of middle pastry bits that have over-puffed. Crumble half of the cheese evenly on each piece of pastry.

4. Top with asparagus, leaving a little gap in the middle then crack an egg into the gaps and reduce oven temperature to 190°C.

5. Bake a further 10–15 minutes until the egg is cooked through. While the tarts are cooking dry fry the prosciutto in a hot frying pan for a minute each side until crispy. Season the tarts with salt and freshly ground black pepper, sprinkle with lemon zest and serve immediately garnished with remaining crumbled cheese, chopped chives and shards of prosciutto.

6. Cook's Note: If you have thick asparagus halve them lengthways, but if they are thin, fine stalks leave them whole.

Prep Time: 40 Minutes

Cook Time: 25 Minutes

Servings: 3

Ingredients

- 8 slices of sourdough
- 4 chorizo sausages, skins discarded
- 200 grams gruyere cheese
- 4 tablespoons fruit chutney
- 50 grams butter
- 8 tomatoes
- 4 eggs
- Salt
- cracked pepper
- fresh parsley, optional

Instructions

1. Preheat the oven to 170°C.
2. Place tomatoes on a lined baking tray and roast until soft and juicy, this should take 20–25 minutes.
3. In a non-stick fry pan over a medium heat, fry chorizo mince until golden and crispy. Chorizo is very fatty so no oil is needed for frying.
4. Place 4 pieces of sourdough on a chopping board. Smear each piece with fruit chutney and top with a slice of gruyere cheese, a large spoonful of chorizo mince

and another slice of cheese. Then, place another piece
of sourdough on top.

5. Melt ½ the butter in a large non-stick fry pan. Place 2
    toasties in the pan and fry on both sides until golden
    brown and cheese has melted. Add the other ½ of the
    butter and fry remaining toasties.

6. Fry eggs in a non-stick fry pan. Season with salt and
    pepper and serve with extra fruit chutney and parsley.

Prep Time: 30 Minutes

Cook Time: 15 Minutes

Servings: 4

Ingredients

- Dry ingredients:
- ½ cup whole wheat flour
- ¼ cup all-purpose flour
- ¼ cup corn starch
- 1 tsp. baking powder
- ¼ tsp. baking soda
- ½ tsp. salt
- 1-2 tsp. sugar, to taste

Wet ingredients:

- 1 cup whole milk + 1 tsp. white vinegar or lemon juice (or just use 1 cup buttermilk)
- 1 large egg
- 1 small overripe banana, mashed (you want ½ cup mashed banana -- if your banana is really big, you might not need all of it)
- 1 TBSP melted coconut oil or vegetable oil
- 1 tsp. vanilla extract

Optional toppings:

- Slices of banana, chopped pecans / walnuts / hazelnuts, chocolate chips, nutella, whatever your heart desires.... and of course maple syrup!

Instructions

1. In a bowl or large glass measuring cup, whisk together all the dry ingredients.
2. In a separate bowl, mash the banana and mix in all the wet ingredients.
3. Add the wet ingredients to the dry ingredients, and mix well to combine. Let the batter sit, without stirring, for 30 minutes. Take a shower, make some tea, and get the waffle iron hot -- just don't skip letting the batter rest! The batter might seem too thin at first, but it will thicken up as it sits.
4. Make waffles according to your waffle iron's instructions. Note: I find with most home waffle irons, it helps to go an extra minute or two after the waffle iron says it's "ready" before removing the waffle if you want a nice, crispy exterior. This will vary depending on your particular machine, so play around with the amount of time it takes to get your waffles to the desired level of crispiness.)
5. Serve immediately with sliced bananas, chopped nuts, and maple syrup. These waffles are best eaten the moment they come off the iron, but if you're set on everyone sitting down to eat at the same time, you can help preserve the crispiness a little by putting cooked waffles directly on the rack in a 150 degree F oven until you're ready to serve.
6. Notes
7. There are plenty of ways to mix up this recipe. Here are some suggestions:
8. For regular waffles: just omit the banana, and increase the oil to ¼ cup. (I like to use 1 tsp. sugar if I'm using a banana, and 2 tsp. sugar if not -- but that's totally personal preference.)

9. To banana bread waffles or regular waffles, try adding a pinch of cinnamon and nutmeg, or other spices like Chinese five spice or ginger.

10. Swap the banana for pumpkin puree and a dash of pumpkin pie spices.

11. Make regular waffles, but stir in a spoonful of cocoa powder to the dry ingredients, and top with chocolate chips. (For add-ins like nuts and chocolate, I prefer to use them as a topping rather than adding them directly to the batter, so I don't have to worry about them burning to the waffle iron.)

12. For quick and easy waffles, I like to make a mix out of the dry ingredients. Just whisk together 5 or 6 times the dry ingredients in a bowl, store in an airtight container, and when you want to make waffles, scoop 1 cup of mix and follow the recipe as written. You can also make smaller or larger batches of waffles easily, just be sure to adjust the wet ingredients accordingly (i.e., for half a cup of mix, halve the wet ingredients).

Prep Time: 30 Minutes

Cook Time: 15 Minutes

Servings: 12

Ingredients

- 1 1/2 cups whole milk
- 1/4 cup white vinegar
- 2 cups all-purpose flour
- 1/4 cup dark brown sugar, packed
- 2 tsp. baking powder
- 1 tsp. baking soda
- 1 tsp. sea salt
- 1 1/2 tsp. cinnamon
- 1 tsp. nutmeg
- 1/2 tsp. ground ginger
- Pinch of cloves
- 2 large eggs
- 1 cup unsweetened pumpkin puree (make your own, here)
- 4 Tbsp. unsalted butter, melted

Optional:

- Chopped pecans, or walnuts, or chocolate chips, to taste
- Maple syrup, butter, whipped cream, etc., for serving
- Or substitute 1 TBSP pumpkin pie spice. If you prefer your pumpkin pancakes plain, go ahead and omit the spices all together.

Instructions

1. To keep finished pancakes warm until serving, pre-heat oven to 200f.
2. In a glass measuring cup or bowl, stir together the milk and vinegar. Set aside to sour while you prep your other ingredients.
3. In a large bowl, whisk together the flour, sugar, baking powder/soda, salt, and spices if using. Try to make sure there are no clumps of brown sugar.
4. In another bowl, combine the buttermilk, pumpkin puree, eggs, vanilla, and melted butter.
5. Add the wet ingredients to the dry ingredients, and mix until just combined – the batter will be lumpy, but that's okay. Over-mixing will cause tougher, gummier pancakes.
6. Place your griddle or skillet over medium-low heat – if you're making the jack-o-lantern flapjacks, you don't want the batter to cook too quickly and burn while you're still making your design. If your using a non-stick surface, do not grease it. If you do oil your pan, use very little.
7. To make the jack-o-lantern faces, pour some of the pancake batter into a plastic squeeze bottle, or an empty (and thoroughly cleaned) ketchup bottle or the like. Onto the griddle or skillet, squeeze two triangles for eyes, and make a mouth; or, draw a spider-web or other design. Once the batter begins to look dry on top, pour or squeeze more batter over your masterpiece. Because your drawing was on the heat first, it will cook longer and turn darker than the rest of the pancake. If you're using nuts, chocolate chips, or other add-ins, sprinkle a small handful on top of the pancake just before flipping. Cook until bubble just barely begin breaking on the surface, and flip your flapjack to reveal

your design! Let cook for another minute or so, or until the underside is lightly browned.

8. Troubleshooting: If the batter in your squeeze bottle is too thick, you can add another tsp or two of milk. If lumps in the batter are clogging the nozzle, you may need to cut a wider opening at the tip. If you pipe your design, and then the image moves around on the pan when you pour more batter on top, your griddle has too much grease on it – wipe it off with a paper towel and try again. If you plan on piping words into your pancakes, remember to write them backwards on the pan, since the image will be mirrored once flipped.

9. It might take a pancake or two to get a feel for how long to leave the batter on the pan to get the right color on it, and you may need to adjust the heat depending on your stove top.

10. Place cooked pancakes onto a plate or tray, and place in the warm oven until ready to serve.

11. Serve with fresh whipped cream, maple syrup, or garnished with more nuts or chocolate chips. Enjoy!

Prep Time: 25 Minutes

Cook Time: 15 Minutes

Servings: 4

Ingredients

- 4-6 large eggs
- 1/3 cup cream
- Sea salt and ground pepper
- 20 grams butter
- ¼ cup natural Greek yoghurt
- ¼ cup good-quality egg mayonnaise
- ¼ cup harissa or kasundi

To serve:

- 4 brioche buns, halved and toasted
- 11/3 cups rocket or spinach leaves
- 12 rashers cooked streaky bacon
- 1 avocado, sliced
- 2 tablespoons purchased dukkah

Instructions

1. I'm not sure if this really needs instructions but here we go! Whisk the eggs and cream together and season with salt and pepper. Heat the butter over a gentle heat in a frying pan and add the eggs. Don't stir for about 30

seconds, then cook, stirring only occasionally, until the eggs are softly set.

2. Whisk the yoghurt and mayonnaise together and swirl through the harissa or kasundi.

3. To Serve: Serve the buns slathered in the spicy yoghurt mix and topped with rocket, bacon, avocado and egg, and finished with a sprinkling of dukkah.

4. Drinks Match: With 'breakfast' and 'brioche', there's nothing better than bubbles. My vote goes to the Hāhā Rōhi Hawke's Bay Sparkling Rosé NV ($20). A mix of merlot, malbec and cabernet sauvignon, it's bold and bursting with berry bagel.

11. Candied Chestnut Cake

Prep Time: 35 Minutes

Cook Time: 15 Minutes

Servings: 5

Ingredients

- 1/4 cup (half stick) unsalted butter, softened
- 1/2 cup (4 oz.) unsweetened chestnut puree (see recipe notes)
- 6 TBSP granulated sugar, separated, plus more for coating the pan
- 4 eggs, separated
- 1 cup, heaping (280g.) candied chestnuts in syrup (see recipe notes above)
- 2 TBSP dark rum (or amaretto, grand mariner, or other flavored liquor)
- 1 tsp. vanilla extract
- 1 cup (107g.) chestnut flour, or hazelnut meal

Pinch of salt

- Confectioner's sugar, for dusting

Instructions

1. Preheat oven to 350f. (176c.). thoroughly grease a 9″ pan, place a round of parchment paper in the bottom, and grease the parchment. Sprinkle the pan with

granulated sugar to coat. (I used a spring-form pan for even easier removal, but I don't think it's necessary).

2. Strain the syrup from the candied chestnuts and reserve it for later – you should have about 1/4 cup of syrup (if you have less than that, add some honey or maple syrup to bring the amount to 1/4 cup). Chop the strained chestnuts and set aside.

3. With a hand or stand mixer, cream together the butter, chestnut puree, and 3 TBSP of sugar. Add the egg yolks one at a time, beating well after each addition. Mix in the chestnut syrup, rum, and vanilla, then fold in the chestnut flour and candied chestnuts. Set aside.

4. Clean your beaters thoroughly, and wipe with a little vinegar or lemon juice to remove any grease. In a separate, clean bowl, beat the egg whites and salt to soft-medium peaks. While beating on high, add the rest of the granulated sugar 1 TBSP at a time and continue to whip until the meringue has reached medium-stiff peaks. (See my post on Angel Food Cake for a visual on meringue peaks.)

5. Fold 1/3rd of the egg whites into the batter to lighten it, then the rest of the egg whites. Mix gently but thoroughly, until no streaks of egg whites are visible.

6. Pour into your prepared pan, and spread the batter to the edges. Bake on the center rack for 25-30 minutes, or until the top turns lightly golden and a tooth pick inserted in the center comes out clean.

7. Remove from oven and let cool completely before removing from the pan. When ready to serve, dust the surface with confectioner's sugar.

Prep Time: 35 Minutes

Cook Time 15 Minutes

Servings: 5

Ingredients

- 1 cup short grain brown rice
- 2½ cups water
- 1 tsp. ground turmeric
- ¾ tsp. fine grain sea salt

For the peanut sauce:

- ½ cup creamy peanut butter (look for one with no sugar added, if you can)
- ¾ cup light coconut milk
- 1½ TBSP fresh lime juice (about half a lime)
- 1 TBSP soy sauce
- 1 tsp. crushed red pepper flakes
- ⅛th tsp. garlic powder
- For the collard rolls (see recipe notes for variations):
- 1 bunch of collard leaves (about 8-10 leaves)
- 1 red bell pepper, cut into thin strips
- 1 english cucumber, cut into thin strips
- 2 large carrots, cut into matchsticks
- 1 or 2 avocados, cut into slices

Handful of sprouts:

- ½-1 cup thinly sliced purple cabbage

Optional: some fresh cilantro, or other herb you like

- Turmeric rice, and peanut sauce

Instructions

For the turmeric rice:

1. Rinse the rice, then place it in a medium saucepan along with the water, turmeric, and salt. Set over high heat, bring to a boil, then cover and reduce the heat to low. Let cook, covered, for about 40 minutes, or until the rice is tender and the water has been absorbed. If the rice is still a little wet when it's finished cooking, remove the lid and let the water evaporate, over low heat, for a minute or two. Do not stir, or the rice will become gluey.
2. Let cool slightly before filling your rolls. Rice can be made in advance. Once cooled, it can be stored in an airtight container in the fridge for up to a week, or portioned into freezer bags and frozen indefinitely.

For the peanut sauce:

1. Mix everything together in a small bowl. If the peanut butter is particularly dry or hard (as natural peanut butters can be if stored in the fridge) microwave for a few seconds to soften, or place in a small saucepan to warm.

For the collard rolls:

2. Get all your veggies and other ingredients (rice, sauce) ready before you begin.

3. Fill a large, shallow skillet (12 or 14 inches) with water, and bring to a simmer. While the water is heating up, fill a large bowl with cool water and add a handful of ice.

4. Wash the collard greens if they are dirty, then dunk one into the boiling water. I like to use the stem as a handle, and just shimmy the leaf back and forth a little to get it submerged. Let the leaf blanch for 20-30 seconds -- it will turn bright green, and soften up so it's easier to roll, and tender enough to eat. Remove from the skillet and plunge the leaf into the bowl of ice water. Repeat with the remaining leaves.

5. When you're ready to roll, pull a leaf out of the bowl and blot it lightly on a clean towel. Spread the leaf onto your counter or cutting board, stem-side-up (the stem forms a large ridge down the back of the leaf). Using a sharp, non-serrated knife, fillet as much of the stem off as you can without cutting through the leaf itself. By this I mean, hold your knife perpendicular to the leaf, and gently slice away as much of the ridge of stem as you can. This will make the leaf more pleasant to eat, and much easier to roll. Slice off the entire stem at the base of the leaf, and flip the leaf over.

6. Add a small amount of each ingredient in a line across the width of the roll, leaving enough room on the sides so you can fold in the sides of the leaf like a burrito. Once all my rice and veggies have been added, I like to add a spoonful of the peanut sauce, too.

7. To roll, fold the bottom of the leaf up over the ingredients, then fold in the sides. Use your fingers to hold the ingredients tight, and roll away from you until the roll is almost closed. You can finish rolling as is, but I like to add a small dab more peanut sauce to the

last little bit of leaf, so that it stick and holds itself shut a little better.

8. Slice the roll in half, and you're done! Repeat with the remaining leaves.

9. Serve with the remaining peanut sauce on the side, for dipping. I like to eat these while the rice is still slightly warm, but they also last really well in an airtight container in the fridge. I've kept them for up to a five days. If the peanut sauce becomes too thick after refrigeration, add a splash of water or coconut milk to thin it out again.

 Prep Time: 1hrs 20 Minutes

Cook Time: 1hrs 35 Minutes

Servings: 6

Ingredients

- 3 TBSP good-quality balsamic vinegar
- 1 TBSP maple syrup
- 1 tsp. dijon mustard
- 1/2-3/4 cup extra virgin olive oil
- pinch of salt, to taste

For the salad:

- 4 firm, not-quite ripe pears (I used bartlett, but use what you like)
- 1 TBSP butter, melted (or coconut oil)
- 1 TBSP dark brown sugar
- 3/4-1 cup walnuts, or pecans
- 8 cups or so of mixed salad greens (I used arugula, spinach, red leaf lettuce, and baby kale, but frisee, radichio, chard, and escarole are all in season in the fall, too)
- 1/4-1/2 cup dried cranberries, or cherries
- 1/4-1/2 cup gorgonzola cheese, or other crumbly blue cheese

Instructions:

For the dressing:

1. Whisk together all the ingredients except the olive oil and salt. While whisking, pour in the olive oil. Start with a half cup, and adjust to taste. Add a pinch of salt, to taste. Cover and place in the fridge until ready to use. Whisk well before using. (Dressing can be made up to a week in advance.)

For the salad:

1. Preheat the oven to 400 degrees F., and line a rimmed baking sheet with aluminum foil or parchment.
2. Cut the pears into wedges (I cut mine into 1/8ths), and remove the stems and cores. Toss with the melted butter and brown sugar, and spread onto prepared baking sheet. Roast for 10-12 minutes, or until just tender (not mushy).
3. Meanwhile, place the walnuts (or pecans) into a dry skillet over medium heat. Toast for 6-8 minutes, or until warm and flavorful. Give the pan a shake, or stir the nuts, every couple of minutes to keep them from burning — keep your eye on them!
4. Combine your mixed greens, dried cranberries (or cherries), and crumbled cheese. When you are ready to serve, add the toasted nuts and roasted pears, while still warm. (You can keep your pears in wedges, as I did, or cut them into bite-sized pieces for easier eating.) Toss with dressing, to taste, and serve immediately.

Prep Time: 16 Minutes

Cook Time 65 Minutes

Servings: 5

Ingredients

- 2-4 TBSP olive oil, or coconut oil
- ½ small yellow onion, diced
- 2-3 cloves garlic, minced
- 1 cup green lentils (brown should work fine as well, but green are what I used)
- 2¼ cups water
- ½ tsp. fine-grain sea salt
- ½ cup rolled oats, processed into flour (or ½ cup storebought oat flour -- make sure the oats are gluten-free if you're gluten intolerant)
- 1 TBSP chia seeds, plus ¼ cup water
- 1 tsp. soy sauce OR gluten-free tamari, for those who are gluten intolerant
- ¼ tsp. crushed red pepper flakes
- ¼ tsp. ground fennel seed
- ¼ tsp. dried thyme
- ¼ tsp. dried oregano
- ¼ tsp. smoked paprika
- ¼ tsp. ground cumin
- ¼ tsp. chili powder
- ¼ tsp. ground black pepper, plus more to taste
- ¼ tsp. kosher salt, or as needed
- ¼ cup fresh parsley, finely chopped

For serving:

- 2-3 large zucchini, spiralized (see recipe notes -- or you can use cooked spaghetti squash, or regular noodle, or any kind of noodle alternative you like)
- your favorite tomato sauce, homemade or store-bought
- Extra fresh chopped parsley, for garnish

Instructions

1. Rinse the lentils and pick over them to make sure there aren't any stones. Drain, and set aside.
2. Place a medium saucepan over medium-high heat, and saute the onion and garlic in 1-2 TBSP oil for about 5 minutes, or until the onion has started to turn translucent.
3. Add the lentils, water, and ½ tsp. salt, and increase heat to high. Bring to a boil, then reduce the heat to maintain a slow, gentle simmer. Let cook for about 30 minutes, or until the lentils are tender with just a little bit of chew. If there is still some water left in the pot when they've finished, drain it off in a strainer. If they start to run out of water and aren't tender yet, add a splash more and keep cooking.
4. While the lentils are cooking, process the oats into flour (to make your own, simply add rolled oats to the bowl of your food processor and blend until finely ground), and mix the chia seeds and water together in the bottom of a large mixing bowl.
5. When the lentils are done, place them in the bowl with the chia seeds, and add in the oat flour and all the remaining ingredients except for the parsley and salt.

Using a potato masher, mash the mixture until most of the lentils are broken up and the mixture is sticky enough to hold together when rolled into balls. If the mixture isn't quite holding together, you can add a TBSP or so of water to help it, or mash a little longer.

6. Add in the chopped parsley and mix to combine. Taste, and adjust seasoning with more salt or spices if needed.
7. Roll the mixture into "meatballs". I used a rounded TBSP to make them all about the same size, and ended up with a little over 20. You can make them bigger or smaller if you like.
8. Add a couple TBSP oil to a large skillet (I like cast iron for this, but nonstick or stainless will work too) and seer the meatballs on all sides until a nice crust has formed (about 2 minutes per side, over medium-high heat). The meatballs should hold together easily, but they are tender so be gently when turning them. I found a pair of silicone-tipped tongs (like these) worked perfectly.
9. Serve directly on top of your favorite sauce, or add the sauce to the pan and coat the meatballs before serving. Serve over zucchini noodles, or other noodly alternative. Enjoy!
10. You can keep zucchini noodles raw, or cook them a bit before serving to warm them up and soften them. Either way, I suggest taking this one extra step before serving up your spiralized zucchini:
11. After spiralizing, place the "noodles" into a large strainer or colander, and sprinkle with a bit of kosher salt. Let them sit for 10-15 minutes (you can do this while the no-meatballs cook) and allow them to drain off their excess liquid. Spread on a clean towel and blot gently before piling into bowls (or quickly sauteing in a hot pan, just for a minute or two) and then serving.

This will help prevent a watery soup from happening in the bottom of your bowl.

12. And because I know some of you are going to ask, this is the spiralizer I use. I've had it for a couple years now, and have been very happy with it so far. It makes quick zoodle dishes and clean up a breeze.

Prep Time: 26 Minutes

Cook Time 45 Minutes

Servings: 7

Ingredients

- 6 large egg yolks (I suggest using pasteurized eggs here, see recipe notes below)
- ½ - ¾ cup granulated sugar, to taste
- 3 cups whole milk
- 1½ tsp. freshly grated nutmeg
- ¼ tsp. cinnamon
- Small pinch of salt
- 1 cup heavy cream
- 1-2 oz. bourbon, cognac, or brandy, to taste (optional)
- 1-2 oz. rum, to taste (optional)
- 1 tsp. pure vanilla extract
- 6 large egg whites + 1 TBSP sugar (optional)
- Whipped cream and freshly grated nutmeg, for serving (optional)

Instructions

1. In a large bowl, or the bowl of your stand mixer, beat the egg yolks until smooth and lightened in color. Add the sugar slowly, while mixing, and continue to beat until pale and fluffy. Set aside.

2. In a saucepan over medium heat, combine the milk, nutmeg, cinnamon, and pinch of salt. Heat until steaming, stirring occasionally. Do not let it boil!

3. Slowly temper the egg with the hot milk mixture. To do this, slowly pour the hot milk mixture into the egg yolks and sugar, while whisking constantly. This will keep the eggs from heating too rapidly and scrambling. Once all of the liquid has been incorporated, return the mixture to the saucepan.

4. Cook over medium-low heat until the mixture begins to thicken slightly, stirring gently but constantly, and scraping the bottom of the pot to prevent scorching. If you have a thermometer, cook until the temperature reaches 160 degrees F. Do not let it boil, or the mixture will curdle!

5. Remove from the heat and stir in the heavy cream, vanilla extract, and liquors (if using -- I typically leave them out, and add them later if I want them). If there are any lumps, pass the eggnog through a fine mesh strainer.

6. Chill in the fridge for at least a couple of hours, or overnight, before serving. Fresh eggnog can be stored for up to a 4-5 days or so, or longer if it has the alcohol added. It should be kept in the fridge at all times. Stir well to mix in any of the nutmeg that may have settled to the bottom before serving, and top with fresh whipped cream and extra nutmeg. Enjoy

Prep Time: 20 Minutes

Cook Time 35 Minutes

Servings: 3

Ingredients

- 4 oz. (by weight) good quality white chocolate, roughly chopped (or about 3/4 cup)
- 2 cups milk (I used whole milk, but I'm sure you could use whatever % you like)
- 3-4 green cardamom pods, crushed
- 1 two-inch strip of orange zest
- 1/2 tsp. pure vanilla extract
- pinch of cinnamon or freshly grated nutmeg, for garnish
- fresh whipped cream, for serving (optional)
- use a vegetable peeler to remove just the outer (orange) part of the rind — try to avoid getting any of the white pith underneath.

Instructions

1. If your chocolate is in a block or a bar, chop it roughly and place it in a large bowl. If it is in chip form, just add it to the bowl as-is.
2. Place a small pot on the stove over medium-low heat, and add the milk, crushed cardamom, and orange zest. Heat until the milk begins to steam, and small bubbles appear around the edges of the pot, stirring frequently

to keep the milk from scorching on the bottom of the pot. As soon as bubbles appear at the edges, remove from the heat — do not let it boil!

3. Place a strainer over the bowl with the chocolate, and pour the milk through to remove the cardamom and orange. Add the vanilla extract, and let sit for 20-30 seconds to allow the chocolate to begin melting. Whisk until smooth.

4. Garnish with a dash of cinnamon or freshly grated nutmeg. Serve as is, or top with a dollop of fresh whipped cream.

Enjoy!

Prep Time: 10 Minutes

Cook Time 50 Minutes

Servings: 9

Ingredients.

- 1 large, or two smaller, kabocha squash (about 4 lbs)
- 2-3 TBSP olive oil, or coconut oil
- 1 medium yellow onion, diced
- 3-4 cloves garlic, minced
- 1½ - 2 tsp. curry powder, to taste*
- ½ tsp. ground cumin
- ½ tsp. ground corriander
- ½ tsp. freshly grated ginger (or ¼ tsp. ground ginger)
- ¼ tsp. ground cinnamon
- ¼ tsp. ground turmeric
- 4-6 cups vegetable stock or water, as needed
- ½ cup full-fat coconut milk, plus more to taste
- Salt, to taste
- Fresh cilantro, for garnish
- Wedges of lime, for serving (optional)

Instructions

1. Preheat oven to 350 degrees F.
2. Remove the stem, and cut the squash into wedges. Scoop out the seeds and stringy insides, and discard them. Place the wedges cut-side up onto a foil lined

baking sheet, drizzle with 1 TBSP olive or coconut oil, and sprinkle with a generous pinch of salt. Roast the squash for 30-40 minutes, or until tender. Remove from the oven and let rest until it is cool enough to handle, then scoop the meat away from the flesh.

3. In a large pot or dutch oven, saute the onion with 1-2 TBSP oil for 5-7 minutes, or until translucent. Add the garlic, curry powder, cumin, cinnamon, ginger, turmeric, and a pinch of salt, and cook for another 1-2 minutes, or until the spices are fragrant.

4. If you have an immersion blender, add the cooked squash and 4-5 cups vegetable stock or water, and puree until smooth, adding more liquid as needed to reach the desired consistency. OR, transfer the cooked onions, squash, and enough vegetable stock or water to blend, to an upright blender and puree until smooth. You may need to do this in batches. Return to the pot and add additional liquid as needed to reach the desired consistency.

5. You can add the coconut milk now, or reserve it for drizzling over the soup later (or add some now, and some later). Add salt to taste, and adjust the level of heat to your liking by adding more curry powder or more coconut milk if needed.

6. Serve with fresh cilantro, and wedges of lime if you'd like a little acidity.

18. Stuffed Portabella Pizzas

Prep Time: 10 Minutes

Cook Time 15 Minutes

Servings: 3

Ingredients.

- 6 large portabella mushrooms
- about ½ cup marinara sauce (storebought or homeade -- I had some in the freezer from our garden last year. This is simply tomatoes, garlic, salt, pepper, and olive oil cooked until thick and saucy.)
- 2-3 oz. shredded mozzarella cheese (or other good melting cheese, or your favorite vegan substitute)
- Toppings (these are just some suggestions -- use any or all that you like. You'll only need a small amount of each for these mini-pies):
- Meats: pepperoni, crumbled sausage or bacon (cooked first), diced ham, shredded chicken
- Veggies: finely chopped green bell pepper, red onion, black olives, chopped artichoke hearts, mini button mushrooms (mushroom on mushroom action!), baby arugula or spinach, etc..
- Other add-on ideas: crushed red pepper flakes, finely chopped fresh basil (optional but recommended), tiny pinch of garlic powder or cajun seasoning, a sprinkling of parmesan cheese, ranch powder, etc.

Instructions

1. Preheat oven to 450 degrees F., and (optionally, for easier clean-up) line a rimmed baking sheet with foil or parchment. Prepare all your toppings and have them at the ready (if you're using meats, cook them and set aside. Chop all your veggies, grate the cheese, etc.)
2. Wipe the surface of the mushrooms clean with a damp cloth, then remove the stems with a paring knife and scrape away the gills using a spoon. The gills are perfectly edible, but removing them will give you more room for stuffing, and help reduce the amount of moisture in the mushrooms.
3. Place the mushroom caps open-side up on the baking sheet, and roast for 12 minutes. Remove from the oven, and gently use a pair of tongs to pick up each mushroom and drain off any moisture that has pooled in it.

4. Return the mushrooms to the baking sheet, and add a small spoonful of marinara sauce to each. Top with a little cheese, and then a small amount of whatever toppings you like. I made some with meat and some without. My favorite was the sausage / green pepper / red onion pizza. (Go figure, these were my dad's favorite pizza toppings, too.)

5. Once the pies are topped, return them to the oven. Let cook for about 5 minutes, or until the cheese is bubbly and golden. If you want, you can switch on the broiler in the last minute or two to get the cheese nice and browned. Once baked, you can add fresh ingredients like baby arugula or chopped fresh basil. Serve.

Prep Time: 15 Minutes

Cook Time 15 Minutes

Servings: 2-3

Ingredients.

- 1 large fillet of arctic char (you can also use other fish like trout or salmon. Look for the freshest fish you can find, and if the fillets are small, use two. My fillet was approx. ½ inch thick x 13 inches long.)
- 1 lb. asparagus, woody ends trimmed off
- 2-3 TBSP olive oil
- 1 meyer lemon, cut into thin slices
- 1 blood orange, cut into thin slices
- a few sprigs fresh thyme, or ½-1 tsp. fresh thyme leaves
- salt and pepper

Instructions

1. Preheat oven to 400 degrees F., and line a rimmed baking sheet with parchment.
2. Spread the asparagus on the baking sheet, drizzle with 1-2 TBSP olive oil, season well with salt and pepper, and toss around the pn to coat evenly. Spread the asparagus into an even layer around the edges of the pan, and lay the fish in the middle, skin-side down.
3. Drizzle the fish with the remaining TBSP olive oil, and season evenly with salt and pepper. Arrange the slices

of citrus on top of the fish, alternating lemon and blood orange slices. scatter the fresh thyme on top.

4. Roast on the middle rack for about 12-15 minutes. Your time will vary depending on how thick your fillet is, and how well done you like your asparagus. I like mine crisp-tender, and using a fillet about ½ inch thick works perfectly for this. To test the fish, prod it gently with a fork in the thickest part. If it flakes and is opaque all the way through, it's done. If necessary, you can remove the fish to a serving patter and return the asparagus to the oven for another minute or two -- or vice versa, if the asparagus is done before the fish. They should be done at about the same time, but again, it will vary depending on the size of your fillet.

5. Remove from the oven and serve immediately. You can eat this as-is, or serve it over a salad (I like arugula here, with its mild peppery flavor) or with a side of rice or other grain for a more filling meal.

Prep Time: 5 Minutes

Cook Time: 30 Minutes

Servings: 3-4

Ingredients.

- 1 head cauliflower
- 3-4 cloves garlic, peeled
- 2-4 TBSP olive oil (plus more for drizzling on later)
- 2 cups dairy free milk of choice (unsweetened), or regular cows milk if you aren't vegan
- 1-2 cups low sodium vegetable stock, or water, as needed
- 1 tsp. fresh thyme leaves
- salt and pepper, to taste

Instructions

1. Preheat oven to 400 degrees F., and (optionally) line a rimmed baking sheet with parchment or foil for easier cleanup.
2. Roughly cut the head of cauliflower into large florets. Discard any green leaves, but leave the core. Dump onto the prepared baking sheet, drizzle with 1-2 TBSP olive oil, and season well with salt. Toss to coat evenly, and spread into an even layer.
3. Place the peeled garlic cloves on a separate, small square of alluminum foil (or you can place them in a small oven-safe ramekin if you prefer not to use foil)

and drizzle with another 1-2 TBSP olive oil. Sprinkle with salt, and if using foil, pull the edges up around the garlic and press to make a pouch around the cloves. Place on the baking sheet along with the cauliflower.

4. Place the tray on the center rack, and roast for about 30 minutes, or until the cauliflower is tender and golden at the edges, and the garlic is fragrant.

5. Transfer the cauliflower and garlic to a small pot, add the milk, 1 cup stock or water, and thyme, and puree using an immersion blender. OR transfer everything to a stand-blender and puree until smooth. Add additional stock/water as needed to reach the desired consistency, and season to taste with salt and pepper.

6. Serve as is, or with a drizzle of good olive oil for garnish. (I also decided to leave a few of the tiniest cauliflower florets on the tray instead of adding them to the soup, and used them to garnish the bowls -- but that's totally optional.)

21. Beet Root Soup

Prep Time: 5 Minutes

Cook Time: 30 Minutes

Servings: 3-4

Ingredients.

- TBSP olive oil
- 2 carrots – roughly chopped
- 1/2 onion – roughly chopped
- 2 cloves garlic – peeled, whole
- lbs. fresh beets, red or yellow
- 2 russet potatoes, roughly chopped
- 1 TBSP balsamic vinegar
- Optional: fresh herbs (such as rosemary, thyme, dill, cardamom...), or some orange juice and zest
- 4 cups water (or vegetable broth)
- Salt and pepper to taste
- Optional: 1 red or yellow beet, shredded

Instructions

2. Wash beets to remove dirt, but do not peel. Remove stem end and cut into halves or quarters. Set aside.
3. Add oil to a large heavy bottom pot over medium-high heat. Add the carrots, onions, and garlic, and saute for 3-4 minutes.

4. Add the beets, potatoes, balsamic, and any whole herbs if using. Add the water and bring to a boil. Cover and reduce heat to medium – cook for 30-40 minutes, or until beets are soft.
5. Puree with an immersion blender, or very carefully transfer in batches to an upright blender and (carefully) blend until smooth. Be extra mindful of spatters with this one, since beets are known for their ability to stain.
6. Season to taste with salt and pepper, and optionally garnish with beet confetti – one beet peeled and grated on a cheese grater.
7. Curried Ginger Rice
8. (Vegan, gluten-free)

9. 2 and 1 TBSP olive oil, separated (or butter/substitute)
10. 1 carrot, diced
11. 1 onion, diced
12. 1 bell pepper, diced
13. Fresh ginger, 1 inch piece, cut into thin matchsticks (or replace with 1/4-1/2 tsp. powdered ginger)
14. 2 cloves garlic, minced
15. 1/2 cup peas
16. 2 TBSP curry powder
17. 2 TBSP cumin
18. 4 cups cooked rice (white, brown, or you could use quinoa or couscous)
19. salt to taste
20. Optional: 1/2 cup raisins or currants
21. Heat 2 TBSP olive oil in a saute pan over medium-high heat. Peel and slice the ginger thinly, then julienne the slices into tiny matchsticks. Add to the hot oil. Add the

carrot and saute for 2-3 minutes. Add the onion, bell pepper, and ginger, and cook another 2-3 minutes.

22. Add the curry powder and cumin to the pan, and let them toast for thirty seconds. Drizzle in 1 TBSP olive oil, add rice, and stir until thoroughly combined.
23. Season with salt to taste, and stir in raisins or currants if using.
24. (Note: this dish is super easy to trouble-shoot. If it's over seasoned, add more rice. If it's not hot enough for you, add more ginger or a dash of cayenne. Too spicy and you can add 1-2 TBSP sugar to mellow it out.)

Prep Time: 5 Minutes

Cook Time: 25 Minutes

Servings: 4

Ingredients.

- 9 oz. package soba (buckwheat) noodles
- 6-8 oz. sugar snap peas, broccoli, or other vegetable (optional)
- 3 TBSP dark toasted sesame oil
- 2 clove garlic, minced
- 2 TBSP fresh ginger, grated
- 1/4 cup rice vinegar
- 1/4 cup soy sauce, or tamari
- 1/4 cup honey (or agave, or sugar)
- 2 tsp. Mirin (sweetened sake)
- 1/4-1/2 tsp. hot chili oil, or to taste (or sriracha, or cayenne pepper)
- 1/2 cup natural creamy peanut butter
- 1/4 cup water, to thin as desired
- Roasted peanuts, for garnish
- Chives or scallions, for garnish (optional)

Instructions

1. In a pan over medium heat, add the toasted sesame oil, garlic, and ginger. If using snap peas or other vegetables, add them to the pan. Saute for 1-2 minutes,

or until the garlic is golden and veggies are bright green. Add the rest of the sauce ingredients, stir until smooth, and thin with water to desired consistency.

2. In a large pot, bring water to a boil. Cook soba noodles according to package directions (usually about three minutes) or until al-dente. Drain, and add to the pan with the sauce and vegetables. Toss to combine. Garnish with roasted peanuts and fresh chives.

Prep Time: 5 Minutes

Cook Time: 5 Minutes

Servings: 1

Ingredients.

- Ingredients per toast -- multiply as needed:
- 1 slice of bread, toasted (I used a whole grain sandwich bread this time, but whatever you like will work -- can be made gluten-free)
- 1 TBSP tahini, or to taste
- 1-2 tsp. honey, or to taste
- 2-3 TBSP pomegranate seeds (arils) -- optional

Instructions

1. Toast bread. Smear with tahini. (Not too much.) Drizzle honey, to taste. Top with pomegranate seeds if you feel like it.

Prep Time: 10 Minutes

Cook Time: 30 Minutes

Servings: 8

Ingredients.

- 2½ cups (10 oz) gluten-free or regular rolled oats, plus extra for sprinkling on top
- 1 tsp. baking powder
- ¼ tsp. baking soda
- ¼ tsp. fine grain sea salt
- ½ cup dairy-free milk (whatever kind you like, or you can use cow's milk if you're okay with it)
- 1 TBSP chia seeds
- 1 cup unsweetened applesauce
- ¼ cup plus 1 TBSP pure maple syrup (preferably grade B or dark amber)
- 1 TBSP coconut oil, melted (plus more for greasing the pan)
- 1 TBSP fresh lemon juice
- ¾ cup frozen wild blueberries

Instructions

2. grey once Preheat oven to 350 degrees F., and grease a non-stick muffin tin (or line it with paper liners). I grease mine using melted coconut oil, but you can use a baking spray if you prefer.

3. In a small bowl, whisk together the milk and chia seeds. Let sit for at least 5-10 minutes while you prepare the rest of your ingredients.

4. In your blender or food processor, add 2 cups (8oz) of the oats. Blend until finely ground and almost flour-like in consistency. Add the remaining oats, baking powder, baking soda, and salt, and pulse once or twice to combine.

5. In a large bowl, stir together the apple sauce, maple syrup, coconut oil, and lemon juice. (Be sure to stir well as you add the coconut oil, so that it doesn't solidify into a solid chunk if your other ingredients are cold.) Add the chia/milk mixture and stir well, making sure there are no clumps of chia seeds.

6. Add the dry ingredients from the food processor to the bowl, and mix to combine. At the very end, add the blueberries and fold them into the batter, stirring as little as possible to avoid staining the batter purple (streaks of purple are fine, but if the whole batter gets tinted they will look baked -- still delicious, just not as pretty).

7. Scoop the batter into your prepared muffin tin. I like to use an ice cream scoop, which does a perfect job evenly dividing the batter, and also gives the muffins a nice rounded top.

8. Sprinkle the top of each muffin with a pinch more oats, then bake on the center rack for 20-25 minutes, or until the muffins are set and the oats on top have started to toast. If your oven heats unevenly, rotate the pan once during baking.

9. Remove from the oven and let cool for 10 minutes before removing from the pan. Once completely cooled, muffins can be kept in an airtight container at room temperature for up to a week, or frozen for up to

a month. (You can thaw them at room temperature, or pop them, frozen, into the microwave for a few seconds. Just be careful if you do, as the blueberries can turn from icy nuggets to bombs of lava surprisingly quickly.)

Prep Time: 35 Minutes

Cook Time: 45 Minutes

Servings: 14

Ingredients.

- 3¾ cups gluten-free rolled oats, plus extra for sprinkling on top
- 1 tsp. phylum husk powder
- 2 tsp. baking powder
- ½ tsp. baking soda
- ¼ tsp. fine grain sea salt
- 1 cup dairy free milk (I like almond milk, but you can use what you like, or sub in regular cow's milk if you aren't vegan)
- 1 TBSP finely ground chia seeds (or 2 TBSP ground flax seeds)
- 4 large, very ripe bananas, mashed (about 2 cups)
- ½ cup pure maple syrup (preferably grade B, but grade A will work, too)
- 3 TBSP coconut oil, melted
- 1 TBSP apple cider vinegar
- 1 tsp. vanilla extract
- 1 cup walnuts or pecans, roughly chopped -- optional (or you can use other add-ins, like chocolate chips, crushed banana chips, coconut flakes, or dried fruit)

Instructions

1. Preheat oven to 350 degrees F., and lightly grease a non-stick muffin tin (using coconut oil, or non-stick baking spray). Set aside.
2. In a bowl or measuring cup, stir together the dairy-free milk and ground chia seeds. (I like to grind my chia seeds myself, using a mortar and pestle or a spice grinder, or you can buy them already ground.) Let sit for at least 5-10 minutes while you prepare the rest of your ingredients.
3. In your blender or food processor, add 3 cups of the oats. Process until the oats are finely ground into an almost flour-like consistency. Add the remaining ¾ cup oats, psyillium husk powder, baking powder, baking soda, and salt, and pulse a couple of times to combine.
4. In a large bowl, mash together the bananas, maple syrup, apple cider vinegar, coconut oil, and vanilla extract. Add the chia/milk mixture and mix well, making sure there are no clumps of chia seeds.. Add the dry ingredients from the food processor, and any nuts or other add INS you choose, and mix until everything is evenly combined.
5. Scoop the batter into the prepared muffin tin, filling each one to just below the rim of the pan. Sprinkle the tops of each muffin with a few extra oats, and bake on the center rack for 20-23 minutes. If your oven heats unevenly, be sure to rotate the pan once during baking.
6. Remove from the oven and let cool for 5-10 minutes before removing the muffins from the pan. They should come out easily. Re-grease the muffin tin, and repeat with the remaining batter. Once completely cooled, muffins can be kept in an airtight container at room temperature for up to a week, or frozen for up to

a couple of months. (I like to pull one out of the freezer and microwave it for about thirty seconds or so. Alternatively, you could thaw frozen muffins in the refrigerator overnight, and reheat them in an oven or toaster oven.)

Prep Time: 30 Minutes

Cook Time: 30 Minutes

Servings: 4

Ingredients.

- 1 cup steel cut oats (look for certified gluten-free if you have a gluten intollerance)
- 3 cups water
- pinch of salt
- For topping (these are all optional, and to-taste):
- fresh or frozen fruit / berries (I used blueberries and raspberries, but any fruit will work)
- a handful of sliced almonds, pepitas, hemp seeds, or other nut/seed (you could even use a little of your favorite granola -- I'm a fan of this Honey & Hazelnut Granola)
- unsweetened kefir, homemade or store-bought
- drizzle of maple syrup, sprinkling of coconut sugar, a few drops of stevia, or any other sweetener you like, to taste

Instructions

1. Add the oats to a small saucepan and place over medium-high heat. Allow to toast, stirring or shaking the pan frequently, for 2-3 minutes.
2. Add the water and bring to a boil. Reduce the heat to a simmer, and let cook for about 25 minutes, or until the

oats are tender enough for your liking. (The oats will thicken up as they cool -- if you prefer them a bit porridge, add a splash more water, or some milk or dairy-free alternative.)

3. Serve with berries, nuts/seeds (or a handful of granola), a splash of kefir, and any sweetener you like, to taste. Dig in

Prep Time: 10 Minutes

Cook Time: 10 Minutes

Servings: 4

Ingredients.

- 1 lb green beans, stems trimmed off
- 1-2 TBSP olive oil
- salt and pepper, to taste (I suggest being fairly generous)

Instructions

1. Preheat oven to 375 degrees F.
2. Spread the green beans into an even layer on a rimmed baking sheet (line with parchment or foil first for easier cleanup, if you wish). Drizzle with olive oil, and sprinkle generously with salt and a bit of black pepper. Toss to coat everything evenly.
3. Place on the center rack, and roast for about 8-10 minutes. I like the green beans to be tender, but still ever so slightly crisp inside. Check them often towards the end, and remove when they've reached your desired level of doneness.
4. Taste, and if necessary add a pinch more salt.

Prep Time: 10 Minutes

Cook Time: 10 Minutes

Servings: 2

Ingredients.

- 2 cups raw almonds
- 2 TBSP coconut oil
- 1 tsp. chili powder (you can use a bit less or more, depending on how strong your powder is)
- 1 tsp, chinese five spice powder
- ½ tsp. fine grain sea salt, or more to taste
- optional: ⅛th-1/4 tsp. cayenne pepper (depending on how hot your chili powder is)
- optional: 1 tsp. coconut sugar, sucanat, or brown sugar, if you want the nuts a little sweeter

Instructions

1. Add oil and nuts to a large skillet, and sprinkle with the spices and salt (you can leave out the cayenne and add it at the end, if you want a little more kick). Set over medium heat and cook, stirring or shaking often, until the nuts have started to darken slightly and smell toasty, about 7-10 minutes.
2. Remove the pan from the heat and sprinkle over the coconut sugar, if using. Taste, and add add cayenne or additional chili powder if you want more heat, while the nuts are still hot. (Keep in mind that the nuts will

have a soft, mealy texture while warm, but will become crunchy again once they've cooled.) Do not add seasoning once the nuts have cooled, or it won't stick. While the nuts are hot, taste for salt and add more if needed.

3. Allow to cool completely. Nuts can be stored in an airtight container at room temperature for up to a few weeks.

Prep Time: 20 Minutes

Cook Time: 25 Minutes

Servings: 5

Ingredients.

- 1 large head of cauliflower
- 1 small bulb of fennel, reserve the fronds
- 2-3 cloves garlic, peeled
- 3-4 TBSP olive oil
- ½ tsp. salt
- 1 1/2 tsp. Whole fennel seeds
- 4-5 cups low sodium vegetable stock
- black pepper to taste
- pinch of cayenne, to taste
- pinch of nutmeg, to taste
- Crushed pistachios and fennel fronds, for garnish
- for a richer, creamier soup, replace 1-2 cups of stock with milk

Instructions

1. Preheat oven to 400 degrees F.
2. Cut the cauliflower in half and remove the core and leaves. Chop roughly into florets, and place in a large bowl.
3. Cut the fronds away from the fennel bulb, and set them aside. Wash the bulb thoroughly, then cut in half and

remove the core, and any outer layers that are loose or damaged. Cut into chunks roughly the same size as the cauliflower florets, and add them to the bowl. Peel the garlic cloves and add them to the bowl.

4. Toss the fennel, cauliflower, and garlic with the olive oil and salt until well coated, and spread on a rimmed baking sheet. Roast for 30-40 minutes, or until tender and cauliflower is browned at the edges.
5. Meanwhile, toast the fennel seeds in a dry pan over medium heat until fragrant and slightly darkened in color. 2-4 minutes, stirring frequently.
6. Add the roasted cauliflower, fennel, and garlic to a large pot along with the vegetable broth and toasted fennel seeds. Puree with an immersion blender until smooth. (Or, transfer the cooked vegetables straight from the oven into your blender, along with the vegetable broth and fennel seeds, and puree until smooth (this should be done in batches). Then pour into a large pot on the stove.)
7. Heat over medium-high until the soup is warmed through. If the soup is too thick, add a bit more stock. Add the cayenne, nutmeg, and salt and pepper, to taste.
8. Serve warm with crushed pistachios and a few sprigs of fennel for garnish.

Prep Time: 1hrs Minutes

Cook Time: 1hrs 10 Minutes

Servings: 8

Ingredients.

- 12 ounces (by weight, or about 2½ cups) hazelnuts, roasted and skinned, plus more for garnish
- 2 tsp. Baking powder
- 6 large eggs, separated, plus 1 whole egg
- ½ cup + 2 TBSP granulated sugar, plus more for coating the pan
- 2 TBSP frangelico liqour (or other flavored liqour, such as amaratto or kahlua, or you can leave it out and use 1-2 tsp. Vanilla extract instead)

Fresh whipped cream:

- 1 cup heavy cream, or double cream
- 1-2 TBSP granulated sugar, to taste
- 1 tsp. good quality pure vanilla extract

Chocolate ganache:

- 3 oz. (by weight, or about ½ cup) dark chocolate, chopped or in chip form
- ¾ cup heavy cream, or double cream

Instructions

For the cake:

1. Preheat oven to 325 degrees F. Lightly grease either two 9 inch pans, or one 9 inch springofrm pan, and add a couple TBSP of granulated sugar. Roll the pan(s) around, so that the sugar coats the bottom and sides evenly. Tap out any excess sugar.
2. In a food processor, pulse together the hazelnuts and baking powder until the nuts are very finely ground. Do not over-blend them, or they'll turn into nut-butter. Set aside.
3. In a large bowl, or the bowl of your stand mixer, whip the egg whites. Once they start to become frothy, gradually add the 2 TBSP granulated sugar, and continue mixing until they have reached medium-stiff peaks.
4. In a separate bowl, beat the egg yolks and whole egg with the remaining ½ cup sugar until pale and fluffy. Add the liquor (or vanilla extract) and ground hazelnut mixture, and stir until fully combined.
5. Using a flexible rubber spatula, fold ⅓ of the eggwhites into the hazelnut and egg yolk mixture. Repeat until all of the eggwhites are incorporated, folding gently until there are no lumps or streaks of eggwhites remaining in the batter.
6. Pour into the prepared pan(s), and place on the center rack of the preheated oven. Bake for about 30 minutes (if using two 9-inch pans) or for 50-60 minutes (if using one 9-inch springform pan), or until the edges of the cake start to pull away from the sides of the pan, and the center of the cake bounces back every so slightly when gently touched.

7. Remove from the oven and let cool completely. If using two cake pans, you can serve each cake individually, or stack them to create a layered dessert. If you made one 9-inch springform pan, you can cut the cake horizontally into two layers (or three thin layers) and fill with whipped cream.

8. Cake can be made in advance, cooled, wrapped in plastic, and kept at room temperature for up to three days. Serve cake with whipped cream, chocolate ganache, and a handful of freshly chopped hazelnuts on top.

For the whipped cream:

1. Combine all the ingredients in a bowl, and whisk (or beat with a hand or stand mixer, or put in a jar and shake) until light and fluffy. Do not over-mix. (Make this right when you are ready to serve.)

For the ganache:

2. Place the chocolate in a bowl. Heat the cream in a small saucepan over medium-low heat until steaming (do not let it boil). Pour the hot cream over the chocolate, and stir until completely smooth and shiny. Ganache can be kept in an airtight container in the fridge for up to the expiration date of the cream. It will become thick like frosting once cooled, and can be rewarmed over low heat, or in ten-second increments in the microwave, until fluid again.